NCLEX: Integumentary System

105 Nursing Practice Questions & Rationales to EASILY Crush the NCLEX Exam!

Chase Hassen
Nurse Superhero
© 2016

Disclaimer:

Highly Recommended Books for Success

NCLEX: Respiratory System : 105 Nursing Practice Questions and Rationales to Easily Crush the NCLEX!
http://amzn.to/1RKLDrR

NCLEX: Endocrine System : 105 Nursing Practice Questions and Rationales to EASILY Crush the NCLEX!
http://amzn.to/237bmFj

NCLEX: Integumentary System: 105 Nursing Practice Questions and Rationales to EASILY Crush the NCLEX!
http://amzn.to/1RVtgCJ

NCLEX: Emergency Nursing : 105 Practice Questions and Rationales to Easily Crush the NCLEX!
http://amzn.to/1V62dIa

EKG Interpretation: 24 Hours or Less to Easily Pass the ECG Portion of the NCLEX!
http://amzn.to/1TylyRo

Lab Values: 137 Values You Know to Easily Pass The NCLEX!
http://amzn.to/1RKM6u2

Fluid and Electrolytes: 24 Hours or Less to Absolutely Crush the NCLEX Exam!
http://amzn.to/2O2zFir

.

TABLE OF CONTENTS

First, I want to give you this FREE gift...

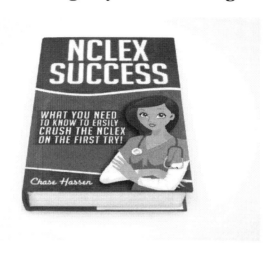

Just to say thanks for downloading my book, I wanted to give you another resource to help you absolutely crush the NCLEX Exam.

For a limited time, you can download this book for FREE.
http://bit.ly/1VvK2e7 .

CHAPTER 1:
NCLEX-RN QUESTIONS, ANSWERS & RATIONALES ON THE INTEGUMENTARY SYSTEM

The following are 105 questions that will help you study for the NCLEX evaluation. All of the questions are based on things you might need to know about the Integumentary System. Compare your answers with the correct answers to see where you may need to study further. Good luck!

1. Name the functions of the skin. Select all that apply.
    a. *Maintenance of a moisture barrier*
    b. *To allow alkalinic secretions to be excreted*
    c. *Protection against microorganisms*
    d. *To act as a mechanical barrier for the body tissues*
    e. *To take in proteins as nutrients for the body*
    f. *To take in fats as nutrients for the body*

Answer: a. c. d. The skin has many functions. It is a barrier mechanically, chemically, and thermally, allowing for acidic secretions to be expressed from the dermis, and acting as a moisture barrier for the body.

2. Heat loss from the skin is dependent upon what?
   a. *The number of sebaceous glands in the skin*
   b. *The blood flow to the skin*
   c. *The number of hair follicles in the skin*
   d. *The ambient temperature*

Answer: b. The blood flow to the skin controls the amount of heat that is lost from the skin. The ambient temperature plays a lesser role in the amount of heat lost from the skin.

3. When heat is excessive, sweat is produced by what glands?
   a. *Eccrine glands*
   b. *Endocrine glands*
   c. *Axillary glands*
   d. *Scalp glands*

Answer: a. During excessive heat, sweat is produced by the eccrine glands in the skin. Eccrine glands are located in most skin areas, including the scalp and axillary area.

4. A client is deficient in a vitamin that is manufactured in the skin. What vitamin is deficient?
   a. *Vitamin A*
   b. *Folic acid*
   c. *Vitamin C*
   d. *Vitamin D*

Answer: d. Vitamin D is manufactured in the skin in response to exposure to sunshine. The other vitamins need to be ingested by the gastrointestinal system.

5. Skin sensation involves which of the following types?
   a. *Pressure*
   b. *Light touch*
   c. *Moisture*
   d. *Vibration*
   e. *Pain*
   f. *Proprioception*

Answer: a. b. d. e. Skin sensation involves detection of pressure, light touch, vibration and pain. Moisture is not a part of skin sensation and proprioception is the ability to detect where a body part is in space without looking at it.

6. The sensitivity of the skin depends upon what?
   a. *The age of the client*
   b. *The gender of the client*
   c. *The density of receptors in the skin*
   d. *The thickness of the skin*

Answer: d. The degree of sensitivity of an area of skin depends on the density of receptors in the skin tissue.

7. The parts of the body considered highly sensitive include the following. Select all that apply.
   a. *Soles of the feet*
   b. *The back*
   c. *The fingers*
   d. *The face*
   e. *The abdomen*
   f. *The buttocks*

Answer: c. d. The fingers and the face have the highest density of receptors and are considered the most sensitive parts of the body.

8. Cells of the skin considered important in cell-mediated immunity are what?
   a. *Islet cells*
   b. *B cells*
   c. *Langerhans cells*
   d. *T-helper cells*

Answer: c. Langerhans cells are specialized skin cells involved in cell-mediated immunity.

9. Oil is produced in the skin by what glands?
   a. *Eccrine glands*
   b. *Apocrine glands*
   c. *Langerhans glands*
   d. *Sebaceous glands*

Answer: d. Oil in the skin is produced by the sebaceous glands. Eccrine glands produce sweat; Langerhans cells are involved in cell-mediated immunity; apocrine glands produce sweat that is potentially malodorous.

10. The outermost layer of the skin is called what?
    a. *The hypodermis*
    b. *The dermis*
    c. *The subcutaneous layer*
    d. *The epidermal layer*

Answer: d. The epidermal layer or epidermis is the outer layer of the skin. Deep to that is the dermis, then the hypodermis, which is also called the subcutaneous tissue.

11. The epidermis is thinnest on what body area?
    a. *The eyelids*
    b. *The fingertips*
    c. *The soles of the feet*
    d. *The back of the hand*

Answer: The epidermis is thinnest on the eyelids, followed by the back of the hand, the fingertips and the soles of the feet in that order.

12. Skin color is determined by what? Select all that apply.
    a. *Sebaceous glands*
    b. *Melanin*
    c. *Carotenoids*
    d. *Oxygenated Blood*
    e. *Deoxygenated Blood*
    f. *Lymph fluid*

Answer: b. c. d. e. Skin color is determined by the melanin, carotenoids, oxygenated blood in arterioles, and deoxygenated blood in the venules.

13. Functions of the dermis include the following. Select all that apply.
    a. *Nerve supply to the skin*
    b. *Contains fibroblasts, mast cells, and macrophages*
    c. *Provides a moisture barrier*
    d. *Contains sweat glands*
    e. *Provides a radiant barrier*
    f. *Contains collagen and elastin*

Answer: a. b. d. f. The dermis contains the nerve supply to the skin. It also contains fibroblasts, mast cells, and macrophages for immunity and the sweat glands. The dermis contains the collagen and elastin that gives skin its elasticity and substance.

14. The part of the skin that provides the most insulation from the hot and cold is what?
    a. *Epidermis*
    b. *Dermis*
    c. *Hypodermis*
    d. *Langerhans cells*

Answer: c. The hypodermis or subcutaneous layer contains fat, which is important in insulation for the body.

15. The thickest areas of hypodermis are located where?
    Select all that apply.
    a. *Back of the hand*
    b. *Sole of the feet*
    c. *Back*
    d. *Fingertips*
    e. *Buttocks*
    f. *Calves*

Answer: c. e. The thickest areas of the hypodermis are located on the back and the buttocks.

16. Eccrine glands are found on which body areas the most?
    Select all that apply.
    a. *Forehead*
    b. *Soles of the feet*
    c. *Back*
    d. *Buttocks*
    e. *Palms of the hands*
    f. *Axilla*

Answer: a. b. e. f. Eccrine glands are particularly found on the forehead, the soles of the feet, the palms of the hands, and the axilla.

17. What is true of the apocrine glands?
    a. *They are the most important glands in sweating.*
    b. *They have the highest concentration in infancy.*
    c. *They do not function until puberty.*
    d. *They release oil onto the skin.*

Answer: c. The apocrine glands are not well understood. They do not function until puberty.

18. Which area(s) of the skin do not have hair follicles?
    a. *The abdomen and the back.*
    b. *The scalp*
    c. *The soles and the palms*
    d. *The buttocks*

Answer: c. Only the soles and the palms are absent of hair follicles.

19. Hair color is determined by what part of the skin?
    a. *The carotenoids*
    b. *The melanocytes*
    c. *The location on the body*
    d. *The age of the skin*

Answer: b. Melanocytes near the hair shaft determine what color the hair coming out of the follicle is.

20. The arrector pili muscles are activated when what happens to the skin?
    a. *A fall in temperature*
    b. *A rise in temperature*
    c. *An increase in sweat*
    d. *Fear*

Answer: a. The arrector pili muscles are activated when the temperature falls, producing classic "goose bumps".

21. Nail growth is slowed by what? Select all that apply.
    a. *Hot weather*
    b. *Illness*
    c. *Increased protein in the diet*
    d. *Cold weather*
    e. *Increased sweating*
    f. *Application of nail polish*

Answer: b. d. Both cold weather and illness will slow the rate of growth of the nails, which normally grow about 0.1 mm per day.

22. The doctor asks the nurse to obtain a culture and sensitivity on a lesion. What does the nurse understand about this procedure?
    a. *It must be done on at least two sites two hours apart.*
    b. *It is generally useless because it only shows skin organisms.*
    c. *It can tell what antibiotics might be helpful when treating the lesion.*
    d. *The wound must be thoroughly cleansed before obtaining the culture and sensitivities.*

Answer: c. A lesion can be cultured and sensitivities to certain antibiotics can be determined so as to find out which antibiotics might be helpful in treating the infection. Only one culture need be taken and the wound must not be cleansed before obtaining the culture.

23. A fungal infection is suspected. What tests can be done to determine the presence of a fungal infection of the skin? Check all that apply.
    a. *Bacterial culture and sensitivities.*
    b. *Blood culture for fungi*
    c. *Fungal culture*
    d. *Wood's light examination*
    e. *Potassium hydroxide exam*
    f. *White blood count*

Answer: c. d. e. Tests for fungal infections of the skin include a Wood's lamp examination, a fungal culture, and a KOH (potassium hydroxide) smear. Bacterial cultures and white blood counts will not show the presence of skin fungi and a blood culture for fungi is likely to be negative.

24. A scabies infection in a child is suspected. What procedure does the nurse do to in order to confirm the infection?
    a. *Check for anti-scabies antibodies.*
    b. *Take a scraping from an area that has been scratched.*
    c. *Take a scraping from an unscratched lesion and look for feces or eggs.*
    d. *Take a scraping and look for the organism living in the tissue.*

Answer: c. To look for the presence of scabies, take a scraping from an unscratched lesion and look for the presence of eggs or feces within the scraping.

25. Common signs of aging skin include what? Check all that apply.
    a. *Xerosis*
    b. *Increased elasticity*
    c. *Increased collagen*
    d. *Decreased subcutaneous fat*
    e. *Seborrheic keratosis*
    f. *Cyanosis*

Answer: a, d, e, Common signs of aging is wrinkling from decreased collagen, decreased elasticity, decreased subcutaneous fat and xerosis or "dry skin".

26. You are seeing a client who has several wheals. You recognize that wheals can come from what sources? Select all that apply.
    a. *A first degree burn*
    b. *A second degree burn*
    c. *An insect bite*
    d. *Hives*
    e. *Angioedema*
    f. *Poison Ivy*

Answer: c. d. e. Wheals are areas of increased edema that can be pale or pink in color. They are often itchy and are caused by insect bites, hives, and angioedema.

27. The client has a rash that involves having multiple vesicles. What can be the cause of these vesicles? Select all that apply.
    a. *Herpes simplex*
    b. *Pemphigus*
    c. *Herpes zoster*
    d. *Second degree burn*
    e. *Scabies*
    f. *Chicken pox*

Answer: a. c. e. f. Herpes infections, scabies and chicken pox can all form vesicles that look like tiny blisters. They can burn or itch.

28. A client has a large area of skin covered by bullae. What are some reasons the client might have this?
    a. *Chicken pox*
    b. *Scabies*
    c. *Contact dermatitis*
    d. *Second degree burns*
    e. *Bullous impetigo*
    f. *Pemphigus*

Answer: c. d. e. f Bullae are large blisters and can be caused by severe contact dermatitis, second degree burns, bullous impetigo or pemphigus.

29. A 16 year-old male client's face is covered in pustules. What do you expect this is from?
    a. *Folliculitis*
    b. *Impetigo*
    c. *Bullous pemphigoid*
    d. *Acne*

Answer: d. Given the age and gender of the client, the most likely cause of the pustules is acne vulgaris. The other choices are less likely and bullous pemphigoid does not include pustules.

30. The client has an area of skin that is made from fibrous tissue that has replaced dermal tissue after an injury. What is this called?
    a. *Collagen band*
    b. *Elastin band*
    c. *Scar*
    d. *Folliculitis*

Answer: c. A scar is an area of skin made from collagen and elastin that replaces damaged dermal tissue.

31. The doctor has asked you to help him do a patch test. What is your understanding of the test?
    a. *It can only be done by doing one patch per day.*
    b. *It differentiates irritant dermatitis from allergic dermatitis*
    c. *The patch must be worn for 12 hours.*
    d. *The presence of erythema and papules is a negative test.*

Answer: b. A patch test is a test where allergens are placed on specially prepared tape and the skin reaction is measured at 48 and 72 hours. Any erythema, papules or vesicles is considered a positive reaction. Several allergen patches can be placed at one time and the patch must be worn for a minimum of 48 hours.

32. A client is scheduled for a punch biopsy. What to you tell the client before the test to educate him or her?
    a. *No anesthesia is necessary as it is such a small area of sampling.*
    b. *The doctor will shave off a piece of skin with a scalpel.*
    c. *The doctor will use a device that punches out a small circle of skin for examination.*
    d. *The doctor will be excising the entire lesion during the biopsy.*

Answer: c. In a punch biopsy, the area is anesthetized and a small device is used to punch out a small circle of skin for pathologic examination. Usually it is not intended to remove the entire lesion and a scalpel is not used.

33. A client is scheduled for a large excisional biopsy. How do you instruct the client before the test?
    a. *Take all medications as prescribed before the test.*
    b. *Coagulation studies should be done on all clients before this type of biopsy.*
    c. *The client should be NPO for 12 hours prior to the biopsy.*
    d. *The client should avoid aspirin or aspirin products for 48 hours before the test.*

Answer: d. Before a large excisional biopsy, the client should refrain from aspirin containing products for 48 hours and should eat a light meal before the biopsy to avoid fainting. Coagulation studies are only recommended if there is a known history of a possible coagulation disorder.

34. Which type of biopsy will definitely require sutures to close it?
    a. *Shave biopsy*
    b. *Excisional biopsy*
    c. *Punch biopsy*
    d. *Skin scraping*

Answer: b. An excisional biopsy is usually large and requires sutures to close the skin defect. A punch biopsy may require one stitch if bleeding does not stop. Shave biopsies and skin scrapings do not require sutures.

35. A client is suffering from severe itching. What are some nursing interventions you should do? Select all that apply.
    a. *Clean the itching areas with antibacterial soap.*
    b. *Apply menthol or camphor to the itching areas.*
    c. *Note the location and degree of the itching as they apply to daily living.*
    d. *Maintain skin hydration.*
    e. *Apply local heat to the affected area.*
    f. *Ask the doctor about prescribing antibiotics.*

Answer: b. c. d. When the patient has itching, take note of the location and degree of itching, maintain skin hydration, and wash the area with mild soap for 14-20 minutes. Apply menthol or camphor to relieve itching. Antibacterial soap is not required and heat will make the itching worse. Antibiotics are not necessary.

36. A client with severe itching from urticaria wants something to control the symptoms. What do you request for the patient?
    a. *A hot water bottle.*
    b. *Diphenhydramine.*
    c. *Systemic steroids.*
    d. *Neosporin*

Answer: b. Diphenhydramine, hydroxyzine or chlorpheniramine are good choices for urticaria. Systemic steroids are a last resort, a hot water bottle will make the itching worse and Neosporin will not be helpful.

37. A client has atopic dermatitis. What other condition(s) might go along with this disorder?
    a. Hives
    b. Allergic rhinitis
    c. Asthma
    d. Impetigo
    e. Patches of painful vesicles.
    f. Bullae

Answer: b. c. Clients with atopic dermatitis can also have asthma and allergic rhinitis, often called the "allergic triad". Hives, impetigo, bullae and painful vesicles are not associated with atopic dermatitis.

38. Common body areas affected by atopic dermatitis include the following. Select all that apply.
    a. The antecubital fossae
    b. The scalp
    c. The backs of the hands
    d. The back of the knees
    e. Fingertips
    f. Eyelids

Answer: a. c. d. f. Areas involved in atopic dermatitis include the antecubital fossae, the back of the hands and top of the feet, the back of the knees, the neck and the eyelids. The scalp and the fingertips are not often involved.

39. The patient has a new diagnosis of atopic dermatitis. What is now indicated?
    a. *Biopsy of the site for confirmation*
    b. *Patch test for allergies*
    c. *Application of witch hazel*
    d. *Hot baths*

Answer: b. If the client has just been diagnosed with atopic dermatitis, a patch test for allergies should be done to diagnose the allergen. A biopsy is not likely to help in the diagnosis. Witch hazel will dry out the skin and emollients should be applied instead. Hot baths should be avoided as the symptoms will intensify.

40. The client with atopic dermatitis understands the nature of his disease when he says what?
    a. *"The doctor said he is giving me medication to cure the disease."*
    b. *"I should take a hot bath every day to relieve my symptoms."*
    c. *"I will not need antibiotics with this condition."*
    d. *"I should keep my fingernails trimmed to avoid scratching the area."*

Answer: d. The client with atopic dermatitis should keep his or her fingernails trimmed short. Hot baths will worsen the condition and topical or oral antibiotics might be necessary if infection is suspected. There is no cure for this condition.

41. Stasis dermatitis is usually found on what body area?
    a. *The lower legs*
    b. *The buttocks*
    c. *The hands*
    d. *The elbows*

Answer: a. Stasis dermatitis is from an excess of edema pooling in the lower extremities. It is not found on the buttocks, the hands or the elbows but is mainly seen in the feet and lower legs.

42. What nursing intervention can best help a client with stasis dermatitis?
    a. *Warm, soapy foot soaks.*
    b. *Giving oral steroids.*
    c. *Raising the legs above the level of the heart.*
    d. *Wearing loose fitting clothing.*

Answer: c. A good nursing intervention for stasis dermatitis is to raise the legs above the level of the heart to improve venous return. Compression stockings can help as well.

43. A client has an itchy rash beneath the face of his watch.
    What does the client likely have?
    a. *Contact dermatitis*
    b. *Folliculitis*
    c. *Atopic dermatitis*
    d. *Herpes zoster*

Answer: a. The patient likely has an allergy to the metal of the back of the watch. This is a type of contact dermatitis. The other conditions are far less likely, especially if the rash exactly matches the shape of the watch face.

44. The client has a new diagnosis of allergic dermatitis.
    What nursing interventions do you perform?
    a. *Teach the client to avoid the allergen.*
    b. *Instruct the client on taking antacids along with oral steroid use.*
    c. *Instruct the client to use topical antibiotic cream on all affected areas.*
    d. *Tell the patient it will almost always spontaneously resolve without treatment.*

Answer: a. A client with allergic dermatitis should learn to avoid the allergen. Oral steroid use is not commonly given unless the condition is severe and antibiotic cream should only be used in areas involved with infection. The dermatitis will not spontaneously resolve as long as the client is exposed to the allergen.

45. Common areas of an intertrigo rash include the following. Select all that apply.
    a. *Beneath the breasts*
    b. *The outside of the elbow*
    c. *The soles of the feet*
    d. *The axillae*
    e. *The perineum*
    f. *The scalp*

Answer: a. d. e. Intertrigo occurs where two skin surfaces are constantly rubbing against one another. This can include the area beneath sagging breasts, the axillae, the perineum, and the antecubital fossae.

46. A common complication of an intertrigo rash is what?
    a. *Impetigo*
    b. *Candida infections*
    c. *Folliculitis*
    d. *Herpes zoster infections*

Answer: b. Candida infections are common complications of an intertrigo rash. The others are not complications of intertrigo.

47. Common nursing interventions for an intertrigo rash include the following. Select all that apply.
    a. *Teach the client to dry the skin carefully.*
    b. *Instruct the client on the application of Neosporin*
    c. *Instruct the client to wear tight fitting clothing*
    d. *Instruct the client on how to apply corn starch to the affected area.*
    e. *Instruct the client to apply talc to dry the skin.*
    f. *Teach the client to use hot soaks to the affected area.*

Answer: a. e. For a client with intertrigo, they should be taught to dry the skin carefully and apply talc to the affected area. Neosporin is not necessary and corn starch can promote infections with Candida albicans. Cool soaks to the affected area should be recommended and the client should wear loose-fitting cotton clothing.

48. A client has just been diagnosed with psoriasis vulgaris. What do you instruct the client as part of client education?
    a. *It is caused by a reaction to nickel.*
    b. *Anxiety and stress can precipitate flare-ups.*
    c. *It is due to an environmental allergy.*
    d. *Steroids can cure the condition.*

Answer: b. Psoriasis vulgaris is an autoimmune disease that can be hereditary. Anxiety and stress can precipitate flare-ups. It is not curable by using steroids and is not related to an allergy or exposure to nickel.

49. Common areas of psoriasis include the following. Select all that apply.
    a. *Palms*
    b. *Soles of the feet*
    c. *Elbows*
    d. *Scalp*
    e. *Abdomen*
    f. *Knees*

Answer: c. d. f. Common areas for psoriasis are the elbows, the knees, the sacral region and the scalp.

50. The client has been placed on anthralin for psoriasis. What nursing education should you give him?
    a. *Apply liberally to all body areas.*
    b. *It is superior to tar shampoos on the scalp.*
    c. *It stains fabric, hair, skin and bathroom fixtures.*
    d. *It is often combined with topical methotrexate.*

Answer: c. Anthralin is a good therapy for psoriasis. It is not often used on the scalp because it stains the hair. It is applied only to affected steroids and is not given with topical methotrexate.

51. The client has been prescribed topical steroids for an outbreak of scalp psoriasis. A nursing intervention could be which of the following?
    a. *Apply a shower cap to enhance the effectiveness of the steroids.*
    b. *Leave the steroids on for 15 minutes and then shampoo.*
    c. *Use anthralin after the steroids have been applied.*
    d. *Tell the patient to apply the steroids on all body areas.*

Answer: a. The effectiveness of steroids is enhanced by applying a shower cap. The steroids do not need to be removed and anthralin is not indicated in scalp psoriasis. Only the lesions should have topical steroids applied to them.

52. The client is on oral methotrexate for psoriasis. What is the most important nursing teaching point that should be made?
    a. *Ultraviolet light is used during therapy.*
    b. *Methotrexate is safe in infancy*
    c. *Use effective birth control in both men and women to avoid chromosomal abnormalities.*
    d. *Take oral methotrexate two hours before a meal.*

Answer: c. When using methotrexate, it is imperative for both men and women to use effective forms of birth control because of the risk of chromosomal abnormalities.

53. A female client has a history of acne vulgaris. What do you tell her about exacerbations of the disease? Select all that apply.
    a. *It is exacerbated by the menstrual cycle*
    b. *It is exacerbated by exposure to UV light*
    c. *It is exacerbated by heat and humidity*
    d. *It is exacerbated by certain facial cleansers*
    e. *It is exacerbated by exposure to cold air.*

Answer: a. c. Acne vulgaris is made worse by the menstrual cycle, by heat and humidity and by excessive sweating. UV light, cleansers and cold air generally do not make acne vulgaris worse.

54. A client asks you how to get rid of his acne. In what ways do you respond? Select all that apply.
    a. *Use medications containing benzoyl peroxide.*
    b. *Use medications containing vitamin A*
    c. *Folic acid will suppress the lesions.*
    d. *Ask the doctor about topical or oral medications.*
    e. *Accutane can be used in severe cases.*
    f. *Cold packs to the face can help.*

Answer: a. d. e. Acne can be treated with benzoyl peroxide used topically, as well as with topical or oral antibiotics. Estrogen can be given to females and Accutane can be used in severe cases. Vitamin A is to be avoided when clients are taking Accutane. Folic acid and cold packs have no effect on acne.

55. A female client has been given a prescription for Accutane for her acne. What is the most important educational piece of information you should give her?
    a. *Use at least two forms of birth control while on Accutane.*
    b. *Accutane may increase the triglycerides.*
    c. *Reduce intake of vitamin A while taking Accutane.*
    d. *Accutane is to be taken with meals to reduce stomach upset.*

Answer: a. Accutane is extremely teratogenic so any female of childbearing age should use at least two forms of birth control while on this medication. It may increase triglycerides and vitamin A should be avoided but these are less important things to know about taking Accutane.

56. A client has acne rosacea. What do you tell the client about the condition? Select all that apply.
    a. *It is associated with having darker skin.*
    b. *It is unaffected by wine intake.*
    c. *It can be worse with exposure to sunshine*
    d. *It can be worse under emotional stress.*
    e. *Spicy foods can make it better.*
    f. *Extremes of temperature can make it worse.*

Answer: c. d. f. Acne rosacea is a chronic skin condition of the face that is worse in people with lighter skin, caffeine, alcohol intake, exposure to sunshine, spicy foods, emotional stress, and extremes of temperature.

57. The treatment of choice for those with acne rosacea is what?
    a. *Oral erythromycin*
    b. *Topical metronidazole*
    c. *Oral tetracycline*
    d. *Accutane*

Answer: b. Topical metronidazole is the treatment of choice for those with acne rosacea.

58. An elderly client at a long term care facility has a new skin tear on the hand. How do you best manage it?
    a. *Contact the doctor so it can be sutured.*
    b. *Trim off the flap of skin that has been torn.*
    c. *Clean the wound and approximate the wound edges.*
    d. *Give a tetanus shot.*

Answer: c. When dealing with an elderly person's skin tear, you should clean the wound, approximate the wound edges, and apply Steri-strips if needed. Cover the wound with gauze for protection.

59. A client is at risk for pressure ulcers. What places on the body should be regularly examined for evidence of these ulcers? Select all that apply.
    a. *Back*
    b. *Sacrum*
    c. *Heels*
    d. *Hands*
    e. *Greater trochanter*
    f. *Ischial tuberosities*

Answer: b. c. e. f. The places most likely to suffer from pressure sores are the heels, sacrum, greater trochanter, and ischial tuberosities.

60. What are some diagnostic tests that need to be done when a client has a deep pressure ulcer? Select all that apply.
    a. *Blood culture*
    b. *Wound culture and sensitivities*
    c. *CBC*
    d. *Bone scan*
    e. *Electrolytes*
    f. *Hematocrit*

Answer: b. d. When a client has a deep pressure ulcer, it should have wound culture and sensitivities done as well as a bone scan to evaluate for the possibility of osteomyelitis.

61. A client has several stage 1 pressure ulcers. What is a good thing to do to avoid furthering these ulcers?
    a. *Giving the client a high carbohydrate diet.*
    b. *Keeping the head of the bed up.*
    c. *Using a donut device to protect the skin.*
    d. *Giving the client a high protein diet.*

Answer: d. A high protein, high vitamin C diet can help pressure ulcers. The head of the bed should be as low as possible and donut devices should be avoided. The client should be instructed to reposition himself/herself every 15 minutes.

62. A family member asks you about their father's stage IV pressure ulcer. What education can you give them?
    a. *Stage IV ulcers usually heal up on their own.*
    b. *Stage IV ulcers may require surgical repair with musculocutaneous flaps.*
    c. *The infection risk is low with proper care.*
    d. *High carb diets can help relieve these kinds of ulcers.*

Answer: b. Stage IV ulcers do not usually heal spontaneously and may require surgical repair with musculocutaneous flaps. The infection risk for these types of ulcers are high. High protein diets are recommended but will likely not treat the problem on their own.

63. A client has an area of broken skin with epidermal and dermal layers only involved in a pressure ulcer. What stage does this represent?
    a. *Stage 1*
    b. *Stage 2*
    c. *Stage 3*
    d. *Stage 4*

Answer: b. The client is suffering from a stage 2 pressure ulcer because only epidermis and dermis are involved.

64. An elderly client has numerous actinic keratoses on his forearms. What do you tell him about these lesions? Select all that apply.
    a. *Some actinic keratoses can become cancerous.*
    b. *Actinic keratoses are hereditary.*
    c. *You can simply peel these off your skin.*
    d. *Actinic keratoses are caused by sun damage.*
    e. *They are more common in dark-skinned individuals.*
    f. *They can turn into melanoma.*

Answer: a. d. Actinic keratoses are seen in light-skinned individuals who have been exposed to the sun. They are not considered hereditary. They can be peeled off but they grow back. They can turn into squamous cell carcinoma of the skin but not melanoma.

65. A good treatment to get rid of actinic keratoses includes what?
    a. Topical 5-fluorouracil
    b. Topical corticosteroids
    c. Oral methotrexate
    d. Oral prednisone

Answer: a. A good treatment for actinic keratoses is twice daily topical 5- fluorouracil. The others are not treatments for actinic keratoses. Topical corticosteroids can be used when there is inflammation from 5- fluorouracil.

66. A client with actinic keratoses asks about medical treatments for the condition. What medical management techniques can you tell him about? Select all that apply.
    a. Cryotherapy with liquid nitrogen
    b. Oral chemotherapy agents
    c. Electrodessication with curettage
    d. Laser excision
    e. Surgical excision
    f. Punch biopsy

Answer: a. c. d. Actinic keratoses can be treated with liquid nitrogen (cryotherapy), electrodessication with curettage, and laser excision. The other choices are not treatments for actinic keratoses.

67. The 88 year old client has a pearlescent, ulcerated bump on his nose. What do you expect it might be?
    a. *Actinic keratosis*
    b. *Squamous cell carcinoma*
    c. *Melanoma*
    d. *Basal cell carcinoma*

Answer: d. The lesion is most likely a basal cell carcinoma based on its pearlescent appearance and ulceration. It is on the nose, which is a frequent area where people get sun damaged skin.

68. A client is diagnosed with cellulitis. What treatment is appropriate?
    a. *An oral antibiotic that covers for Staphylococcus pyogenes.*
    b. *Topical Neosporin*
    c. *Oral antibiotics that cover for Gram negative bacteria.*
    d. *Topical methotrexate*

Answer: a. Cellulitis is highly likely to be caused by Staphylococcus pyogenes so an antibiotic that has Staph penetration would be appropriate.

69. Complications of cellulitis include which of the following? Select all that apply.
    a. *Gangrene*
    b. *Folliculitis*
    c. *Bullous pemphigus*
    d. *Sepsis*
    e. *Abscess*
    f. *Atopic dermatitis*

Answer: a. d. e. Common complications of cellulitis if left untreated include abscess formation, sepsis and gangrene.

70. Your client has been diagnosed with cellulitis. What is the most important thing you can do to prevent cross-contamination on the floor?
    a. *Give prescribed antibiotics.*
    b. *Thorough hand washing.*
    c. *Wear a mask when treating the client.*
    d. *Use droplet precautions.*

Answer: b. Thorough hand washing and standard precautions can help prevent cross-contamination between the patient and others on the floor. Antibiotics treat the infection but take a while to reduce contamination. A mask and droplet precautions are not necessary in this situation.

71. You are selecting staffing for your shift. You have a client with herpes zoster. Who do you select to take care of the client?
    a. *An LPN who had Herpes zoster last year.*
    b. *A pregnant RN.*
    c. *A new RN who has never had chicken pox before.*
    d. *A LPN who is on immunosuppressant medications.*

Answer: a. Herpes zoster is a manifestation of having had the chicken pox virus before. The logical choice would be to have the LPN who had herpes zoster in the past because this is a person who has had known chicken pox in the past. Since you don't know the status of the pregnant nurse and you know a nurse has never had the chicken pox before, these would be riskier choices. An LPN who is immunosuppressed is at a higher risk of becoming infected with the chicken pox virus, especially if she hasn't had the chicken pox before.

72. A client has suffered a thermal burn. Which factors determine the depth of injury? Select all that apply.
    a. *Length of exposure to fire*
    b. *Body surface area involved*
    c. *Location of burn*
    d. *Temperature of fire*
    e. *Length of time until treatment*

Answer: a. d. The temperature of the fire and length of exposure determine the depth of the injury in a thermal burn.

73. Extent of burn in an electrical burn is related to what factors? Select all that apply.
    a. *Duration of contact*
    b. *Type of electrical wire*
    c. *Voltage*
    d. *Type of current*
    e. *Pathway of current*
    f. *Tissue resistance*

Answer: a. c. d. e. f. In an electrical burn, the degree of injury depends on duration of contact, type of current, voltage, pathway of current and tissue resistance to the current. The type of electrical wire has no effect.

74. The client has a diagnosis of impetigo on the face. What treatment is indicated?
    a. *Topical Neosporin*
    b. *Antibiotic that covers for Streptococcal species*
    c. *Antibiotic that covers for Staphylococcus aureus*
    d. *Antibiotic that covers for Gram negative bacteria*

Answer: c. Impetigo is caused by Staphylococcus aureus. Antibiotics that cover for Staphylococcus aureus tend to be best for impetigo.

75. A diabetic client has a large carbuncle on the upper back.
What are some treatments that can be used for this
condition? Select all that apply.
   a. Topical Neosporin
   b. Warm Moist soaks
   c. Incision and drainage
   d. Systemic coverage for Staphylococcus aureus
   e. Topical bacitracin
   f. Washing with a strong soap

Answer: b. c. d. Treatments for carbuncles include applying warm moist soaks to bring the carbuncle to a head, incision and drainage, and systemic coverage for Staphylococcus aureus. Topical antibiotics tend not to help this condition and washing may prevent recurrences but does not treat the condition.

76. A client has just been diagnosed with Herpes zoster.
What can you provide them in the way of client
education?
   a. Herpes zoster is not contagious
   b. Herpes zoster can lead to months or years of pain.
   c. Herpes zoster is a secondary complication to the measles.
   d. Herpes zoster usually occurs on the face.

Answer: b. Herpes zoster is a secondary function of having the chicken pox virus. It can cause chicken pox to those who have never had chicken pox. Two-thirds of clients have herpes zoster on the trunk. Post-herpetic pain can last for months or years.

77. Immunosuppressed clients or those in severe pain from Herpes zoster can be given what form of treatment?
    a. *Tylenol with codeine*
    b. *Atarax (hydroxyzine)*
    c. *Immune boosters*
    d. *Acyclovir (Zovirax)*

Answer: d. Acyclovir (Zovirax) can be given to clients who are immunosuppressed or who are in severe pain to shorten the duration of the disease. Tylenol with codeine and Atarax can help control some of the symptoms.

78. A medication given to prevent outbreaks of herpes type 2 (genital herpes) include what?
    a. *Topical acyclovir*
    b. *Oral Valtrex (valacyclovir)*
    c. *Atarax*
    d. *Vicodin*

Answer: b. Oral Valtrex (valacyclovir) can be given prophylactically to prevent outbreaks of genital herpes. The other treatments can be used for symptoms or for treatment of active disease.

79. A client asks you about warts. What do you tell them?
    a. *Warts are caused by many different viruses and bacterial infections.*
    b. *Warts appear different depending on the body area involved.*
    c. *There is no treatment for warts.*
    d. *Warts cannot cause cancer.*

Answer: b. Warts are caused by human papillomavirus and look different, depending on the body area involved. There are several topical treatments for warts, including cryotherapy and burning of warts. Cervical warts can increase the risk of cervical cancer.

80. What can be said of genital warts? Select all that apply.
    a. *They are not highly contagious.*
    b. *They are spread through sexual intercourse.*
    c. *Genital warts can cause cervical cancer in women.*
    d. *They are caused by a single virus.*
    e. *They are more common in men than in women.*

Answer: b. c. Genital warts are contagious and are spread through sexual intercourse. They can be seen equally in men and women. They are caused by many different strains of human papillomavirus and put women at risk for cervical cancer.

81. Ringworm of the body is also called what?
    a. *Human papillomavirus infection*
    b. *Tinea cruris*
    c. *Tinea pedis*
    d. *Tinea corporis*

Answer: d. Ringworm of the body is called tinea corporis. Tinea pedis is fungal foot infection and Tinea cruris is also called "jock itch". It is not caused by human papillomavirus.

82. A client has been diagnosed with tinea cruris. What patient education information can you give?
    a. *It is more common in women.*
    b. *It does not spread easily.*
    c. *It is often treated with topical miconazole.*
    d. *It rarely itches or burns.*

Answer: c. Tinea cruris is a fungal infection more common in men than in women. It is highly contagious and is often treated with topical miconazole. The main symptoms are itching and burning.

83. A client has been diagnosed with scabies and you are asked to educate them about the condition. What do you say?

    a   Itching is very severe.
    b   It is most common on the scalp.
    c. It is caused by a fungus.
    d. It is a self-limited disease.

Answer: a. Scabies is an infection from a skin mite. It is most common on the nipples, gluteal folds, waistline and arms/hands. It requires treatment in order to affect a cure. The most common symptom is severe itching, which can lead to excoriation and secondary infections.

84. A family you have been seeing as a community nurse has had a child infected with scabies. How do you educate the family? Select all that apply.

    a. *Treat the victim of the disease and any other family members who have symptoms.*
    b. *Use a scabicide such as Kwell applied to the entire body for 8-12 hours.*
    c. *It is not necessary to wash bedding.*
    d. *Change bed linens every day.*
    e. *It is not very contagious among adults.*

Answer: b. d. Scabies is highly contagious. Treat all family members with Kwell for 8-12 hours on the entire body even if they have no symptoms. Wash all clothing, bedding, and bath towels in hot water at the same time. Change bed linens every day until the infection is gone.

85. Pediculosis can involve what body areas? Select all that apply.
    a. Scalp.
    b. Body.
    c. Soles of feet.
    d. Palms of hands.
    e. Groin.

Answer: a. b. e. Pediculosis can involve the scalp, body and groin area. Different types of lice are responsible for the different body areas involved.

86. You are advising a family that has had an outbreak of Tinea capitus. What do you tell them as a way of educating the family? Select all that apply.
    a. Apply a topical pediculicide like Kwell or Rid to the scalp of all family members.
    b. Only one treatment is necessary.
    c. Wash or dry clean linens and clothing.
    d. Disinfect combs and brushes.
    e. Treat all school children exposed to the lice.
    f. Vacuum all carpets and upholstery.

Answer: a. c. d. f. Apply a topical pediculicide to all family members but school contacts need only to be assessed for lice. They need to retreat the infestation in 8-10 days. Wash or dry clean all linens and clothing and disinfect combs and brushes. Vacuum all carpets and upholstery.

87. A client has a large area involved in a second degree burn. What is a hallmark sign of second degree burns?
    a. *Blisters*
    b. *Red, shiny skin*
    c. *Black or gray skin*
    d. *Itching*

Answer: a. The hallmark sign of a second degree burn is blistering of the skin. Reddened skin is seen in first degree burns and black or gray skin is seen in third degree burns. Second degree and first degree burns can itch as they are healing but this can be seen in either type of burn.

88. A thermal burn that affects the bone is called what?
    a. *First degree burn*
    b. *Second degree burn*
    c. *Third degree burn*
    d. *Fourth degree burn*

Answer: d. A thermal burn affecting the bone is called a fourth degree burn.

89. A good way to assess a patient for the presence of inhalational injuries following a fire include what? Select all that apply.
    a. *Check the nares for burns of the hairs inside the nose.*
    b. *Check a carboxyhemoglobin level.*
    c. *Listen to the chest for rhonchi.*
    d. *Check cardiac/pulse rate.*
    e. *Check for stridor.*
    f. *Inspect the oropharynx.*

Answer: a. b. d. e. f. All of the above ways are good ways to assess for the presence of inhalational injurie following a fire except listening for rhonchi of the lungs.

90. The most important thing to do when a patient has been exposed to an acid on their skin is what?
    a. *Flush with sodium bicarbonate solution, which is basic and will counteract the acid.*
    b. *Flush with KOH solution.*
    c. *Remove all clothing.*
    d. *Flush with copious amounts of water.*

Answer: d. With any kind of chemical burn, flushing with copious amounts of water is important. It is not necessary to flush with an alkaline solution, which may trigger a thermic response. Removing affected clothing should be part of the treatment but removing all clothing is secondary to flushing the area immediately.

91. The most important first aid fact in dealing with a client who has sustained an electrical burn is what?
    a. *Flush burned areas with copious amounts of water.*
    b. *Shut off the electrical source before approaching the client.*
    c. *Monitor the airway.*
    d. *Provide O2 by nasal cannula.*

Answer: b. Before approaching the client, make certain the electrical source of the injury is shut off. The airway should be monitored and the patient given 100 percent O2 by mask. Most electrical burns do not need to be flushed with water.

92. You are treating a client in a burn unit with severe burns. Which care is most appropriate?
    a. *Intramuscular Demerol for pain.*
    b. *IV morphine sulfate for pain.*
    c. *Give oral medications on schedule.*
    d. *Give subcutaneous heparin to avoid DVT.*

Answer: b. Clients with severe burns should not have intramuscular or subcutaneous injections. At least 2 IV sites are necessary with IV morphine sulfate given for pain. Oral medications should be avoided because of a risk of aspiration or ileus.

93. In the acute phase of burn care, what nursing intervention is most appropriate?
    a. *Instructing the family not to visit until the client is more stable.*
    b. *Keeping the room cool.*
    c. *Monitor for clinical manifestations of sepsis.*
    d. *Giving pain medication when the client complains of pain.*

Answer: c. In treating someone with an acute burn, monitor for sepsis and teach the family how to wear protective gear to prevent infection. The client is at risk for hypothermia so keep the room warm. Pain medication should be given on a scheduled basis so as to stay on top of the pain.

94. Nutritional support is important for acute burn clients because:
    a. *Oral intake is often low because of gastrointestinal concerns.*
    b. *High protein is necessary for wound healing.*
    c. *Fluid losses can be high.*
    d. *Metabolic rates are 100 percent higher than normal.*

Answer: d. Nutritional support in the acute burn clients because metabolic rates are 100 percent higher than normal.

95. Wound care for third degree burn care involves the following. Select all that apply.
    a. *Premedication for pain before debridement procedures.*
    b. *Showering or spraying the wounds.*
    c. *Providing soap and water to wounds daily.*
    d. *Dry dressings to wound areas.*
    e. *Loosening tissue with scissors or forceps during or after hydrotherapy.*
    f. *Application of occlusive dressings after wound care.*

Answer: a. b. e. For third degree wound care, the client should be premedicated for pain before debriding. Debriding can involve hydrotherapy by showering, spraying or tubbing the patient. Loosen dead tissue with scissors or forceps to enhance debridement. Soap and water are not necessary for these wounds. A wet to dry dressing is appropriate to enhance debridement.

96. The best way to prevent contractures in burn patients is to do what?
    a. *Use ace wraps around the joints.*
    b. *Allow freedom of movement of the arms and legs.*
    c. *Place burned areas in anti-contracture positions using splints.*
    d. *Provide psychological support.*

Answer: c. To prevent contractures, the burned areas should be placed in anti-contracture positions using splints with early occupational and physical therapy. The patient should be encouraged to use the arms and legs but burned areas are likely to be under-used in the healing process so contractures can still happen.

97. For fourth degree burns, the best method of treatment is what?
    a. *Donor grafts until healing has progressed enough for autograft treatment.*
    b. *Full thickness grafts involving skin and soft tissue to cover bone.*
    c. *Split-thickness skin grafts from an unburned area of the body.*
    d. *Secondary healing until an autograft can be placed.*

Answer: b. In a fourth degree burn, bone is involved so excision of the burned area followed by full thickness grafting using skin and soft tissue to cover exposed bone.

98. In teaching about those at risk for burns, the nurse notes that these groups of people are at a high risk of burns:
    a. *Children under the age of 4.*
    b. *School-age kids*
    c. *Adolescents*
    d. *Middle aged individuals*
    e. *The elderly*

Answer: a. e. Children under the age of 4 and the elderly at are the highest risk of burns.

99. Circumferential burns of the thorax are particularly
    dangerous because:
    a. *They can restrict chest excursion.*
    b. *They are at a particularly high risk of infection.*
    c. *They involve too large an area to graft.*
    d. *They are often associated with inhalation injury.*

Answer: a. Circumferential burns of the thorax are
particularly dangerous because they can contract, restricting
chest excursion.

100.   Compartment syndrome of the upper extremity is
        usually caused by what?
    a. *A burn that extends to the bone*
    b. *A circumferential forearm burn*
    c. *A second degree burn to the shoulder on the same
        side*
    d. *A third degree burn to the proximal forearm*

Answer: b. Compartment syndrome of the upper
extremity is caused by a circumferential forearm burn that
contracts and restricts the circulation and nerve supply to the
hand.

101. A nurse is caring for a client with a facial burn in the acute phases. What is the most important nursing intervention?
   a. *Counseling the patient on self-esteem following a facial burn.*
   b. *Nutritional support*
   c. *Observation for inhalation injury*
   d. *Observation for infection*

Answer: c. In the acute phase of a facial burn, the most important nursing task is to observe for the possibility of inhalational injury.

102. Dietary concerns in a client with severe burns includes which of the following?
   a. *Giving enteral feedings until bowel sounds return.*
   b. *Providing a high protein and high carb diet in the early stages of the burn.*
   c. *Instituting a high lipid enteral feeding as soon as possible.*
   d. *Giving solid food along with extra fluids by IV in the early stages.*

Answer: a. It is important to give enteral nutrition in the early stages of a burn in case of ileus and to wait until bowel sounds return before attempting a high protein, high carb diet.

103. What parameters are important when dealing with a patient in the burn unit? Select all that apply.
   a. *The client should secrete a minimum of 30 cc of urine per hour.*
   b. *The client should have a systolic blood pressure above 120.*
   c. *The client should have a systolic blood pressure below 140.*
   d. *The client should have normal sodium and potassium*
   e. *The client should have a body temperature of 96 degrees or above.*
   f. *The client should have a body weight within 30 percent of pre-injury weight.*

Answer: a. d. The client should have a minimum urine output of 30 cc per hour, a BP of greater than 90 systolic, a normal sodium and potassium, a temperature of 98 degrees or above and a weight within 10 percent of pre-injury weight.

104. In the prehospital care of burn victims, what takes priority?
   a. *Prevention of infection*
   b. *Removal from source of the burn*
   c. *Evaluation for compartment syndrome*
   d. *Evaluation for poor self-esteem*

Answer: b. In the prehospital phase, the priority item is removing the client from the source of the burn.

105.   Activities needed to be done in the rehabilitative
    phase of burn care include these. List all that apply.
    a.   *Reconstructive surgeries*
    b.   *Physical therapy*
    c.   *Wound debridement*
    d.   *Observation for infection*
    e.   *Electrolyte balance*
    f.   *High protein diet*

Answer: a. b. In the rehabilitative phase of burn care, the
emphasis is on reconstructive surgeries and physical therapy
and less on electrolytes, diet, infection and wound
debridement.

CONCLUSION

I hope you received a ton of value from this book. Remember, practice makes perfect so you may need to repeat these questions.

If you enjoyed this book, would you be kind enough to leave a review on Amazon? Your reviews can help others to see what kinds of helpful resources are out there!

Thank you and good luck on your medical endeavors! I'll talk to you soon and see you in the next book!

- Chase Hassen

Nurse Superhero .

Highly Recommended Books for Success

NCLEX: Cardiovascular System : 105 Nursing Practice and Rationales to Easily Crush the NCLEX!
http://amzn.to/1MaIcxI

NCLEX: Emergency Nursing: 105 Practice Questions and Rationales to Easily Crush the NCLEX!
http://amzn.to/1qrnPlN

Lab Values: 137 Values You Know to Easily Pass The NCLEX!
http://amzn.to/1qrnPlN

EKG Interpretation: 24 Hours or Less to Easily Pass the ECG Portion of the NCLEX!
http://amzn.to/1q2GS5o

Fluid and Electrolytes: 24 Hours or Less to Absolutely Crush the NCLEX Exam!
http://amzn.to/237wWJV

NCLEX: Endocrine System : 105 Nursing Practice Questions and Rationales to EASILY Crush the NCLEX!
http://amzn.to/1oxMjZd

NCLEX: Respiratory System : 105 Nursing Practice Questions and Rationales to Easily Crush the NCLEX!
http://amzn.to/1oxMHqq

Made in the USA
Middletown, DE
04 September 2024